Adaptative Immunity in Echinodermata

Adaptative Immunity in Echinodermata

Michel Leclerc

ELIVA PRESS

Published by Eliva Press
Email: info@elivapress.com
Website: www.elivapress.com

ISBN: 978-1-63648-226-2

Contents

Innate and adaptative immunity in the sea-star Asterias rubens 3

Abstract... 3

INNATE IMMUNITY. 3

MATERIAL AND METHODS.. 4

RESULTS. 4

RESULTS 5

CONCLUSION 6

CONCLUSION 10

RESULTS 10

DISCUSSION AND CONCLUSION 11

REFERENCES... 11

THE SEA STAR IGKAPPA GENE AND NEW CONCEPT 12

Abstract:... 12

INTRODUCTION.. 12

MATERIAL AND METHODS:... 12

RESULTS 13

DISCUSSION CONCLUSION... 16

References 16

MHC genes CLASS I, CLASS II IN INVERTEBRATES:
THE ECHINODERMATA 17

Abstract.. 17

INTRODUCTION.. 17

MATERIALS AND METHODS... 19

RESULTS 19

CONCLUSION 22

NEW CYTOKINE GENES IN AN INVERTEBRATE: THROMBOXANE ONES IN
ECHINODERMATA.EVIDENCE OF PLATELETS................................... 24

INTRODUCTION.. 24

MATERIALS AND METHODS:..24

RESULTS 25

1 Evidence of Platelets in Echinodermata...25

DISCUSSION AND CONCLUSION: 26

2 Evidence of Platelets in Echinodermata...26

REFERENCES:..27

BENCE-JONES PROTEIN, RAT IGG, H.R.P , ALKALINE PHOSPHATASE,

BOVINE SERUM ALBUMINE(BSA) USED AS ANTIGENS IN THE IMMUNE

RESPONSE OF THE SEA STAR...28

INTRODUCTION..28

MATERIALS AND METHODS...28

RESULTS 29

DISCUSSION CONCLUSION...29

References 30

Innate and adaptative immunity in the sea-star Asterias rubens

Dr Michel Leclerc,
Université d'Orléans

Abstract: The axial organ of the sea star Asterias rubens is a primitive immune organ. The B-like cells, when stimulated by various antigens, produce antibody substances correlating with Mouse Ig Kappa genes. On the other hand elements of the innate immunity are present in Asterias rubens such as Toll-like receptors, interleukin receptors, complement components which contribute to initiate the « antibody factor »

A large number of investigations performed in the last few years, in our Laboratory, have provided evidence that the sea star Asterias rubens (echinoderma) posseses a primitive immune system with cellular and humoral responses functionally similar to those of the immune system of vertebrates. It appears that all the elements necessary to these responses are present in the axial organ, which can then be considered as an ancestral lymphoid organ. Two main population of cells are present in this organ: phagocytic cells and cells that are morphologically and functionally similar to the lymphocytes of vertebrates. When isolated axial organ cells were stimulated "in vitro" by a variety of antigens, a soluble factor was secreted in the culture medium, that specifically lysed sheep red cells sensitised with the corresponding antigen (ref 1). This lytic reaction required the presence of thermolabile factor (complement) present in mammal serum. Moreover, it could be demonstrated that this antibody factor was produced by the B-like cell but only when T-like and phagocytic cells were present during the antigenic stimulation.

A detail review of these findings has already been published. (ref 1 and 2) We have observed that the antibody factor showed some homologies with human kappa-like(ref 3) and correlated with Mouse Ig kappa precursor genes (ref4).

INNATE IMMUNITY.

We have also observed that the sea-star A.rubens present a panel of Toll-like receptor genes.When compared to other Invertebrates and because the immune function of Toll in Drosophila was not then known...It was assumed that TIL (now known as TLR1) might participate in mammalian development. However, in 1991, it was observed that a molecule, with a clear role, in immune function in mammals: the interleukin-1 (IL-1) receptor (found also in sea-star), had homology to drosophila Toll, the cytoplasm portions of both molecules were similar (ref 5)

Always in drosophila, in 1997 TLR4, as an LPS sensing receptor was discovered.

TLR4 plays a role for initiating an adaptive immune response (ref 6). On the other hand, Toll-like receptor genes have been recently discovered in the sea-urchin (ref 7) In the present paper, we have analysed the Toll-like receptor genes of the immunized sea-star Asterias rubens and the control ones.

MATERIAL AND METHODS

Immunization was performed on 20 sea-stars, in an aquarium with sea water at 10°c by using Horse - radish peroxydase (HRP) (Sigma Products) as antigen at a concentration of 1mg/ml. 20 non -injected animals were used as controls. The axial organs were removed; RNA was extracted, using Trizol(Invitrogen) according to manufacturer instructions, from immunized sea stars(HRP) and controls(C). cDNA was normalized using double strand specific nuclease essentially as described by Zhulidov et al (ref 8). cDNA was fragmented using DNA Fragmentase (New England Biolabs), according to the manufacturer's instructions. After ligation of adapters for illumina's GSII sequencing system, the cDNA was sequenced on the illumina GSII platform sequencing 1x 100 bp from one side of the approximately 200 bp fragments. Sequences were assembled using Velvet (Zerbino et al(ref 9) 2007).

RESULTS.

First results concern significative Toll-like receptor genes found in immunized sea-stars

I)HRP(Immunized animal):**TLR13_MOUSE Toll-like receptor 13 and TLR 12 MOUSE TLR-Like receptor(homologies of 63% with mouse).**
Second results concern Toll-like receptors found in control sea-stars(non-immunized):
-TLR1 Toll-like receptor1
-TLR4 Toll-like receptor 4
-TLR3 Toll-like receptor 3
-TLR5 Toll-like receptor 5
-TLR7 Toll-like receptor 7
-TLR9 Toll-like receptor 9

CONCLUSION:

Genes playing a key role in the innate immune system as TLR1 or TIL are present in A.rubens and Strongylocentrotus purpuratus (sea-urchin) .TLR4 was also found in Drosophila(ref 6), A.rubens, and, TLR3, TLR5, TLR7, TLR9. We must notice that only the sea-star (among Invertebrates) presents TLR12 and TLR13 genes, after immunization .We have to say that the sea-star immune model remains enigmatic in terms of immunization.

Finally, an effective innate immune system is already present in Echinoderma as shown in sea-urchin (ref 10) and sea-star and in Invertebrates like in Insects.

Innate immunity: cytokins

Non-adherent-nylon wool cells(T-like subpopulation) can release soluble lymphokine-like mediators, after stimulation with P.W.M sepharose 6 MB beads, with mitogenic properties(ref 11). Some interleukins were discovered in 1997 (ref 12)such as IL1.

RESULTS

We describe first « interleukin genes » then « interleukin receptor genes » as compared to mammals.

a) Control - « Nuclear factor interleukin-3-regulated protein »:

The results of our BlastX (Blast Version 2.2.20, Parameters: -e 0.001 -F F -b 3 -v 3 -I T -a 16 -m 7) were the following.

One contig (NODE_3558_length_451_cov_24.356985) could be annotated via BLASTX to mouse "Nuclear factor interleukin-3-regulated protein" from the SWISSPROT database, with an e-value of 2.87689e-10. On an aligned region of 62 amino acids, 42 positive and 28 identical amino acids were found.

b)HRP - « Nuclear factor interleukin-3-regulated protein »:

One contig (NODE_48893_length_689_cov_15.156749) could be annotated via BLASTX to mouse "Nuclear factor interleukin-3-regulated protein" from the SWISSPROT database, with an e-value of 1.49652e-09. On an aligned region of 57 amino acids, 40 positive and 26 identical amino acids were found.

We study now the interleukin 1 and more specially interleukin 1 receptors:

a)Control - « X-linked interleukin-1 receptor accessory protein-like 2 »:

One contig (NODE_21299_length_1163_cov_23.764402) could be annotated via BLASTX to mouse "X-linked interleukin-1 receptor accessory protein-like 2" from the SWISSPROT database, with an e-value of 2.64154e-07. On an aligned region of 278 amino acids, 110 positive and 60 identical amino acids were found.

b)HRP - « X-linked interleukin-1 receptor accessory protein-like 2 »:

One contig (NODE_23687_length_300_cov_7.280000) could be annotated via BLASTX to mouse "X-linked interleukin-1 receptor accessory protein-like 2" from the SWISSPROT database, with an e-value of 7.2295e-05. On an aligned region of 77 amino acids, 38 positive and 27 identical amino acids were found.

And now the interleukin-1 receptor-associated kinase 4:

a)Control - « Interleukin-1 receptor-associated kinase 4 »:

One contig (NODE_45921_length_271_cov_7.907749) could be annotated via BLASTX to mouse "Interleukin-1 receptor-associated kinase 4" from the SWISSPROT database, with an e-value of 0.000100449. On an aligned region of 96 amino acids, 37 positive and 22 identical amino acids were found.

b)HRP - « Interleukin-1 receptor-associated kinase 4 »:

No contig matched.

We finish with the interleukin-17 receptor B as compared to mammals:

a)Control - « Interleukin-17 receptor B »:

One contig (NODE_31878_length_179_cov_15.167598) could be annotated via BLASTX to mouse "Interleukin-17 receptor B" from the SWISSPROT database, with an e-value of 0.000617054. On an aligned region of 42 amino acids, 24 positive and 14 identical amino acids were found.

b)HRP - « Interleukin-17 receptor B »:

One contig (NODE_46091_length_308_cov_16.399351) could be annotated via BLASTX to mouse "Interleukin-17 receptor B" from the SWISSPROT database, with an e-value of 0.000279731. On an aligned region of 49 amino acids, 28 positive and 16 identical amino acids were found.

As shown, it exists also an Interleukin-17 receptor A:

a)Control - « Interleukin-17 receptor A »:

No contig matched.

b)HRP - « Interleukin-17 receptor A »:

One contig NODE_13602_length_446_cov_23.168161) could be annotated via BLASTX to mouse "Interleukin-17 receptor A" from the SWISSPROT database, with an e-value of 0.000671577. On an aligned region of 81 amino acids, 38 positive and 24 identical amino acids were found.

CONCLUSION

The immunization leads to modifications in the case of « Interleukin-1 receptor-associated kinase 4 » and in the case of « Interleukin-17 receptor A » where this last appears in immunized animals. Furthermore interleukin genes(most of them corresponding to interleukin receptor genes) such as IRPL2, IRAK 4, IL-17RB, IL-17RA are present in the sea-star Asterias rubens.

How to explain this phenomenon? To try to interprate it could be a challenge as compared to mammal interleukins. Nevertheless these observations would indicate that certain interleukins and particularly « receptors »recalling mammal ones are present in the immune system of the sea star.

We note specially, in mammals that, the interleukin 17 receptor B is implicated in the immune response by mediating the activation of NF-Kappa B; that the interleukin 17 receptor A belongs to a novel family of inflammatory cytokines. As for the IRAK 4, it is required for various responses induced by Il-1R and toll-like receptor signals

Innate Immunity: complement components.

In earlier results, complement-like activity, was found in another sea-star: Asterias forbesi (ref.13). As for Asterias rubens, observed in it genome, we can say:

At first, Components of the classical pathway as compared to mammals, were discovered:

in a)Control - Complement C1q subcomponent subunit A:

One contig (NODE_55223_length_184_cov_8.456522) could be annotated via BLASTX to mouse "Complement C1q subcomponent subunit A" from the SWISSPROT database, with an e-value of 8.55742e-06. On an aligned region of 72 amino acids, 29 positive and 25 identical amino acids were found.

b)HRP - Complement C1q subcomponent subunit A:

No contig matched, no hit was found. Then,

a)Control - Complement C1q subcomponent subunit B:

One contig (NODE_48557_length_161_cov_19.316771) could be annotated via BLASTX to mouse "Complement C1q subcomponent subunit B" from the SWISSPROT database, with an e-value of 8.55742e-06. On an aligned region of 57 amino acids, 33 positive and 19 identical amino acids were found.

b)HRP - Complement C1q subcomponent subunit B:

One contig (NODE_68235_length_178_cov_7.724719) could be annotated via BLASTX to mouse "Complement C1q subcomponent subunit B" from the SWISSPROT database, with an e-value of 3.97232e-10. On an aligned region of 44 amino acids, 39 positive and 28 identical amino acids were found.

Then

a)Control - Complement C1q subcomponent subunit C:

One contig (NODE_37343_length_278_cov_12.356115) . On an aligned region of 39 amino acids, 25 positive and 19 identical amino acids were found.

b)HRP - Complement C1q subcomponent subunit C:
Three contigs could be annotated via BLASTX to mouse "Complement C1q subcomponent subunit C" from the SWISSPROT database. The best contig (NODE_29181_length_277_cov_7.790614) with an e-value of 3.67148e-09. On an aligned region of 45 amino acids, 27 positive and 22 identical amino acids were found.

We observe now the C2 Component:
Five contigs could be annotated via BLASTX to mouse "Complement C2" from the SWISSPROT database. The best contig (NODE_23089_length_519_cov_15.136802) with an e-value of 7.65302e-07. On an aligned region of 153 amino acids, 59 positive and 38 identical amino acids were found. And now what about the component C4?
a)Control - Complement C4-B:

One contig (NODE_95392_length_215_cov_10.818604) could be annotated via BLASTX to mouse "Complement C4-B" from the SWISSPROT database, with an e-value of 3.48532e-06. On an aligned region of 76 amino acids, 40 positive and 21 identical amino acids were found.

b)HRP - Complement C4-B:
One contig (NODE_58696_length_164_cov_11.884147) could be annotated via BLASTX to mouse "Complement C4-B" from the SWISSPROT database, with an e-value of 7.51259e-05. On an aligned region of 44 amino acids, 26 positive and 21 identical amino acids were found.

Then, we see the C3 component which is central, in mammals, to both the classical and alternative pathways:

a)Control - Complement C3:
Seven contigs could be annotated via BLASTX to mouse "Complement C3" from the SWISSPROT database. The best contig (NODE_25262_length_1200_cov_21.958334) with an e-value of 3.2395e-49. On an aligned region of 355 amino acids, 128 positive and 173 identical amino acids were found.

b)HRP - Complement C3:
Eleven contigs could be annotated via BLASTX to mouse "Complement C3" from the SWISSPROT database. The best contig (NODE_15219_length_398_cov_19.402010) with an e-value of 4.96748e-24. On an

aligned region of 146 amino acids, 79 positive and 59 identical amino acids were found.It must be noted that C3 belongs to, also, the ALTERNATE pathway.
We give now the obtained results concerning the components of the membrane-attack complex as compared to mammals.

We begin with the very important C9:
a)Control - Complement component C9.
Three contigs could be annotated via BLASTX to mouse "Complement component C9" from the SWISSPROT database. The best contig (NODE_46472_length_143_cov_10.104895) with an e-value of 1.41746e-05. On an aligned region of 31 amino acids, 17 positive and 15 identical amino acids were found.

b)HRP - Complement component C9:
No contig matched, no hit was found.

Then we look about the C5 component:
a)Control - Complement C5:
One contig (NODE_75605_length_236_cov_32.677967) could be annotated via BLASTX to mouse "Complement C5" from the SWISSPROT database, with an e-value of 0.000634854. On an aligned region of 55 amino acids, 27 positive and 19 identical amino acids were found.

b)HRP - Complement C5:
Two contigs could be annotated via BLASTX to mouse "Complement C5" from the SWISSPROT database. The best contig (NODE_7717_length_665_cov_13.831579) with an e-value of 6.42528e-17. On an aligned region of 212 amino acids, 99 positive and 57 identical amino acids were found.

At last we observe the C8 Component:
a)Control - Complement component C8 alpha chain:
Twelve contigs could be annotated via BLASTX to mouse "Complement component C8 alpha chain" from the SWISSPROT database. The best contig (NODE_68667_length_311_cov_10.845659) with an e-value of 6.7995e-15. On an aligned region of 95 amino acids, 33 positive and 42 identical amino acids were found.

b)HRP - Complement component C8 alpha chain:
Six contigs could be annotated via BLASTX to mouse "Complement component C8

alpha chain" from the SWISSPROT database. The best contig (NODE_43169_length_2163_cov_11.209893) with an e-value of 6.36046e-14. On an aligned region of 45 amino acids, 42 positive and 33 identical amino acids were found.

CONCLUSION

The main components of Complement as compared to mammal ones were found in the sea star: How genes are expressed? By which pathway (direct or alternative pathway)? It could be a working hypothesis which needs to be explored. However, it is said that in immunized animals, no hits were found with C9 and C1q (subcomponent subunit A):it remains enigmatic. It could be expected that the sea-star specific immune reaction needs all these genes to be expressed.

Adaptative Immunity: « The antibody factor »
Two main populations of cells are present in the axial organ : phagocytic cells and cells that are morphologically and functionnaly similar to the lymphocytes of vertebrates (Fig 1) .In cooperation with the sea-star complement, they initiate the "antibody factor" (ref 14) Recently kappa genes were discovered in the sea-star A.rubens (ref.4). We now present the DNA structure of these genes in immunized and control sea-stars.

RESULTS

We recall that antibody factor was isolated and purifiied(ref 14). In 2000, it was shown that it presented homologies with human kappa-like (ref 3). Using the same approach(ref.4), the sea-star genomes(Asterias rubens, Patiria miniata°) were analysed.
In Asterias rubens:
One contig(Immunized sea-stars) (NODE 13406 length 132 cov 46.075756) could be annonated via BLASTX to mouse "e kappa chain V-III region MOPC 63" from the SWISSPROT database, with an e-value of 0,000458269.(Fig 2). On an aligned region of 39 amino acids, 21 positive and 16 identical amino acids were found.
Otherwise,it was shown that:
One contig(controls) (NODE_1857_length_169_cov_25.875740) could be annotated via BLASTX to mouse "IG KAPPA CHAIN V-V REGION MOPC 41" from the SWISSPROT database, with an e-value of 0.000886447.(Fig 3) On an aligned region of 33 amino acids, 17 positive and 11 identical amino acids were found.
In Patiria miniata° also, Ig kappa chain V.III region MOPC 63,
Ig kappa chain region MOPC 41 and Ig kappa chain V-V region K2 were detected in a significant manner.

DISCUSSION AND CONCLUSION

These observations confirm that certain mammal structures are present in the immune system of the sea star, and this finding strongly supports the idea that an effective immune system is already present in the sea-star: A.rubens. The main acquisition of Echinoderms seems to be the cellular differentiation in two subpopulations of cells, ancestral to T and B lymphocytes, and their interplay with phagocytes resulting in the synthesis of specific humoral antibody factor. Although all efforts to find a primitive form of immunoglobulin in sea-urchin genome(ref 7) have been unsuccessful, it is the first time, we present arguments indicating that vertebrate immunoglobulin Kappa genes are present in an invertebrate and Deuterostomes. It appears that the antibody factor has a molecular weight of 120-130.000 daltons(ref14) with 4 sub-units of 30.000 daltons each: it could be composed of 4 « kappa chains ».In conclusion the "Avenir" of the immune sea-star study is a bright one.

REFERENCES

1.Brillouet, C,Leclerc,M.,Luquet,G. Cell. Immunol. 84, 138-144 (1984)

2.Leclerc, M.,Brillouet,C.,Luquet, G. Bull. Inst. Pasteur
84, 311-330 (1986)

3.Leclerc,M., Eur. J. Morph. 38, 206-207(2000)

4.Leclerc,M, Dupont,S.,Hernroth, Immunol.Letters.138, 197-98 (2011)

5.Gay,N.J.,and Keith, F.J. Nature. 6325, 351-355 (1991)

6.Medzhitov, R., Preston-Hurlburt,P.,Janeway,C.A.Nature.,6640,388-394 (1997)

7.Rast,J.P.,Smith,L.C.,Loza-Coll, M.Science.314,952-956(2006)

8.Zhulidov P.A.,Bogdanova,E.A, Shcheglov, A.S. Nucleic.Acid. Res.3, 32-37 (2004)

9..Zerbino D.R and Birney,E. Genome Research. 18, 821-829(2007)

10.Hibino,T.,Loza-Coll,M.,Messier,C. Dev.Biol.300 (1) 349-365 (2006)

11.Leclerc,M.,Brillouet,C.,Luquet,G.,Scand.J.Immunol.,14,281-284(1984)

12.Legac,E.,Vaugier,G.L, Bousquet,F.,Scand.J.Immunol.,44,375-380(1997)

13.Leonard,L.A., et al Dev.Comp.Immunol.14,19-30 (1990)

14.Delmotte,F.,Brillouet,C.,Leclerc,.M Eur.J.Immunol.16, 1325-1330 (1986)

° Patiria miniata Genome studied under the direction of Pr. E.Davidson. (2012) U.S.A

THE SEA STAR IGKAPPA GENE AND NEW CONCEPT

By Michel Leclerc

556 rue Isabelle Romée, 45640 SANDILLON, Immunology of Invertebrates, France

Abstract:

Next to the sea star T and B lymphocytes, the preservation of the IgKappa gene for so extended a period of evolution in organisms as distinctively different as sea star, fish, mammal, indicates that it plays an essential rôle in the survival of organisms: rôle in the regulation of immune response, in Asterids. The presence of Fc receptor gene, Fab gene in Asterias rubens, MHC genes corroborate these data.

Key-words:Invertebrates ; Asterids;IGKAPPA genes.

INTRODUCTION.

The purpose of this work is to draw attention to the mass of Igkappa genes that has accumulated on the sea star Immune system since 2011. From this year, genomes of immunized and non-immunized sea stars to HRP (horse-radish peroxydase) have been studied (1). Although IgKappa gene has been isolated (2) and found in mouse, this gene has also been detected in fish (Zebra fish and Larimiththys crocea) and mammals.In this paper we will mainly review information on a fish : Larimiththys crocea and a mammal :Tupaia chinensis, to attempt to evoke Igkappa gene evolutionary considerations .

MATERIAL AND METHODS:

Immunized and non-immunized Asterias rubens sea stars to HRP were used (1). The axial organs were removed; RNA was extracted using Trizol(Invitrogen) according to manufacturer instuctions from immunized sea stars (HRP) and controls (C).

cDNA was normalized using double strand specific nuclease essentially as des cribed by Zhulidov et al (3).cDNA was fragmented using DNA Fragmentase (New England Biolabs), according to the manufacturer's instructions. After ligation of adapters for Illumina's GSII sequencing system, the cDNA was sequenced on the Illumina GSII platform sequencing 100 bp from one side of the approximately 200 bp fragments. Sequences were assembled using Velvet Zerbino et al.(4)

Assembled nodes were used for further assembly including *Beta vulgaris* EST-Data from NCBI in MIRA.

12

RESULTS

First result concern non-immunized animals i-e controls and contig to Larimichthys crocea (fish) :

-One contig (Contig3054|m.205) could be annotated via BLASTX to Larimichthys crocea "Ig kappa chain C region" from the TREMBL database, with an e-value of 3.415e-09. On an aligned region of 102 amino acids, 46 positive and 29 identical amino acids were found.

Second one is obtained from immunized sea stars to HRP Another contig (Contig12275|m.10416) could be annotated via BLASTX to Larimichthys crocea "Ig kappa chain C region" from the TREMBL database, with an e-value of 2.538e-09. On an aligned region of 90 amino acids, 42 positive and 24 identical amino acids were found.

At last, we discover transcriptomes of contigs via BLASTX to the mammal : Tupaia chinensis

a) in : controls

CCCGCTGAGTTTTTGAAACATATTGCCAAGTTAAAATATCTCATACCCTAAT
AATACACC
ATGTAATGTATTGCTTTAACATTGTAAAGATCAATGTGTGTACTACTGTAGTT
AATATAT
CAGATCTCTCTGAAGTTAACACGTGTATCATACTTCATGGAGGCATGCACCT
CAGCCTTG
GTTATCCCTTGGGAAAAGTTCTGTAAGAGTAGAATTGTGTACCAGTGGGAC
TAAACATAA
TTGTGTGCATCTGTTTGGATAATATAAAAATAATATTTTACAATGTGAAAGTA
TTTGTCA
AGTGCATGGTGTTAGGAAAATTAAAAAGACTACATTTGTTTTTCTGTTTTGT
TACCTTTG
CAATAAGTGTTATGACACTGTTGGAAACAATAAAATGTTCAAATTTTGTTAT
A 3'

b) Second in immunized sea stars to HRP :

One contig (Contig12017|m.10218) could be annotated via BLASTX to Tupaia chinensis "Ig kappa chain V-III region HAH" from the TREMBL database, with an e-value of 3.11e-09. On an aligned region of 68 amino acids, 43 positive and 25 identical amino acids were found.

TGATGAATCTCTTAAAATTATATTTAAAAATTACAAATTAAAAATTATTTGAT
AT
TTTGTTCTGGCTCAAACCTTATTGTATTTTGTGTTGTATCAAGACTATGTGCC
TGGACTTGGTTT
GGGATCTTGCACCCCTAGGGTGGTTCTGTGGGGAACCGTGACAAGTGTTT
CTGGAGGAAC
TTTTGTGAGAATTGTAGAAGAACACAAGTGAACCTCATGAACAAAGCAAA
CACCCACTTT
GTCAGAGATAGATTATCCTGTTCACAAATATCACAGTTATGCAGGTGTTTTT
TGTTTTTT
TTCAATCTTTGTCTTTTTCAGACATTTATGGCAATGCAGTCCAAGTATGCAC
AACCAATG
TTTGTTTGTGGTAAATCTTTGTATGAAAACTATGTGTTTATTCACACTGTGAT
ATCTACT
TAGTAAATTCATTCAATTTTCAGGGTTGATGCTTTGTAAACTTTGCTTTTTGT
ATAAAAT
AAGGAAACATAAATGGAATGTGAGGTAAAACAAAGTCAACAATGTACATA
AATGTGGCCA
AGTCACACTAATGGGTTAAAAGATAACTTTGTAAATGAGGCGTGAGACAA
ATGTAACTTT
TTTGTCGCAGTCTTTTCCTGTACATTCAAAAGCTGTTCATGATTTTTCATTG
CAAAAATA
AATAAATTGACCTTAAGAAGTTACAAGGTCATATATTACTACAAAACCACGT
TCCCCTCA
TATGTTACTCTTTTGTGCACATCAGTGTAGAACCACCCACATATGTATATTGC
GCCACTG
ACCTATGACATTTGATGAATGCAATCGATGTGTAACACTTGTGGAATATTG
AAGTGTGT
GTAGTACAATGGCACATTGTCCGTGTTTTGTATAAAAATAGGAAATAAAATG
GTACACCA
CT 3'

There is evidence for the presence of Igkappa genes through the animal kingdom. These results are summarized in table I and Table II :

-Contig3054|m.205
tr|A0A0F8CMX3|A0A0F8CMX3_LARCR Ig kappa chain C region
OS=Larimichthys crocea GN=EH28_01288 PE=4 SV=1

- Contig3376|m.6635
tr|L9JQR9|L9JQR9_TUPCH Ig kappa chain V-III region HAH OS=Tupaia chinensis
GN=TREES_T100021693 PE=4 SV=1

- Contig15579|m.12525
tr|L8HL23|L8HL23_9CETA Ig kappa chain V-III region SIE (Fragment) OS=Bos
mutus GN=M91_06423 PE=4 SV=1

- TR38397|c0_g1_i1|m.2857
tr|A0A0F8C094|A0A0F8C094_LARCR Ig kappa chain V-I region Wes
OS=Larimichthys crocea GN=EH28_01990 PE=4 SV=1

- TR48242|c0_g3_i1|m.3430
tr|A0A091ENA6|A0A091ENA6_FUKDA Ig kappa chain V-VI region NQ2-6.1
(Fragment) OS=Fukomys damarensis GN=H920_01478 PE=4 SV=1

TABLE 1: The Igkappa genes in controls.

And now, what about immunized sea stars to HRP, ?

- Contig12017|m.10218
tr|L9JQR9|L9JQR9_TUPCH Ig kappa chain V-III region HAH OS=Tupaia chinensis
GN=TREES_T100021693 PE=4 SV=1(similar protein)

- Contig12275|m.10416
tr|A0A0F8CMX3|A0A0F8CMX3_LARCR Ig kappa chain C region
OS=Larimichthys crocea GN=EH28_01288 PE=4 SV=1

- Contig8150|m.7973
tr|A0A0F8CMX3|A0A0F8CMX3_LARCR Ig kappa chain C region
OS=Larimichthys crocea GN=EH28_01288 PE=4 SV=1

- Contig18903|m.13528
tr|L8HL23|L8HL23_9CETA Ig kappa chain V-III region SIE (Fragment) OS=Bos
mutus GN=M91_06423 PE=4 SV=1

- Contig12300|m.10433
tr|A0A091DDJ6|A0A091DDJ6_FUKDA Ig kappa chain V-V region T1

15

OS=Fukomys damarensis GN=H920_10033 PE=4 SV=1

- Contig11501|m.9857
sp|P01841|KAC5_RABIT Ig kappa-b5 chain C region OS=Oryctolagus cuniculus

TABLE II : The Igkappa genes in HRP (from immunized sea stars to HRP)

DISCUSSION CONCLUSION

The sea star Igkappa gene is clearly the oldest IgKappa gene of the immune system of animals.

It shows already two Ig sites ! The forms of Igkappa genes are all found in vertebrates, they share many details with the sea star, including the presence of Ig sites.

The preservation of the Igkappa gene in immunized and non-immunized sea stars is an excellent opportunity for further experiments.It is important to notice that the Igkappa chain V-III region HAH of Tupaia chinensis is situated (in the assumptions behind the theory of evolution) between the Igkappa chain precursor V-II region (RPMI/133) and Igkappa chain precursor V-IV region/121.

The preservation of the IgKappa gene for so extended a period of evolution in organisms as distinctively different as sea star, fish, rodent, mammal, indicates that it plays an essential rôle in the survival of the organisms, rôle in the regulation of the immune response.

Additionally, the existence of members of the IgKappa gene family with conserved functional characters, indicate that the sea star IgKappa gene has evolved prior to the evolutionary divergence between Invertebrate and Vertebrates : It must be claimed.

On the other hand, the discovery of a Fc receptor gene, of a Fab gene, MHC genes, in Asterias rubens genome, corroborate the presence of the primitive Invertebrate antibody in asterids (**IPA**) (**5**).(6)

References :

1)Leclerc M, et al. Immunol Lett 2011 ;138(19):7-198.
2) Vincent N, et al. Metagene 2014 ; 2 : 320-322
3)Zhulidov PA, et al. Nucleic Acid Res 2004 ; 3 : 32-37
4)Zerbino DR, et al. Gen Res 2007;18 : 821-829
5)Leclerc M, Amer.J.Immunol 2013 94-95
6)Leclerc M, et al Int.J.Biotech Bioeng 2(1):37-38
DICUSSION

MHC genes CLASS I, CLASS II IN INVERTEBRATES: THE ECHINODERMATA

by Michel Leclerc

556 rue Isabelle Romée, 45640 SANDILLON (FRANCE)

Abstract: For the first time MHC Class I and ClassII genes were described in Echinodermata, (Invertebrates).
HLA-DRB1, HLA -DQB1 genes from Class II; HLA-E, HLA-B genes from Class I have been found in genomes of Ophiocomina nigra(Ophuirids) and Antedon bifida (Crinoïds): Two Echinodermata which present the IPA (Invertebrate Primitive Antibody).

Key words: Invertebrates; Echinodermata; MHC genes

INTRODUCTION:

As C.A Janeway wrote in 2001 (Ref 1) :

"The function of MHC molecules[1] is to bind peptide fragments derived from pathogens and display them on the cell surface for recognition by the appropriate T cells[2]. The consequences are almost always deleterious to the pathogen—virus-infected cells are killed, macrophages are activated to kill bacteria[3] living in their intracellular vesicles, and B cells are activated to produce antibodies that eliminate or neutralize[4] extracellular pathogens. Thus, there is strong selective pressure in favor of any pathogen that has mutated in such a way that it escapes presentation by an MHC molecule.

Two separate properties of the MHC make it difficult for pathogens to evade immune responses in this way. First, the MHC is polygenic[5]: it contains several different MHC class I and MHC class II genes, so that every individual possesses a set of MHC molecules[6] with different ranges of peptide-binding specificities. Second, the MHC is highly**polymorphic**; that is, there are multiple variants of each gene

---

[1] https://www.ncbi.nlm.nih.gov/books/n/imm/A2528/def-item/A3065/
[2] https://www.ncbi.nlm.nih.gov/books/n/imm/A2528/def-item/A3278/
[3] https://www.ncbi.nlm.nih.gov/books/n/imm/A2528/def-item/A2622/
[4] https://www.ncbi.nlm.nih.gov/books/n/imm/A2528/def-item/A3100/
[5] https://www.ncbi.nlm.nih.gov/books/n/imm/A2528/def-item/A3153/
[6] https://www.ncbi.nlm.nih.gov/books/n/imm/A2528/def-item/A3065/

17

within the population as a whole. The MHC genes are, in fact, the most polymorphic genes known

Because of the polygeny of the MHC, every person will express at least three different antigen-presenting[7] MHC class I molecules and three (or sometimes four) MHC class II molecules on his or her cells. In fact, the number of different MHC molecules[8] expressed on the cells of most people is greater because of the extreme polymorphism of the MHC and the codominant[9] expression of MHC gene products.

The term polymorphism comes from the Greek *poly*, meaning many, and *morphe*, meaning shape or structure. As used here, it means within-species variation at a gene locus, and thus in its protein product; the variant genes that can occupy the locus are termed alleles. There are more than 200 alleles of some human MHC class I and class II genes, each allele being present at a relatively high frequency in the population. So there is only a small chance that the corresponding MHC locus on both the homologous chromosomes of an individual will have the same allele; most individuals will be heterozygous[10] at MHC loci. The particular combination of MHC alleles found on a single chromosome is known as an MHC haplotype[11]. Expression of MHC alleles is codominant[12], with the protein products of both the alleles at a locus being expressed in the cell, and both gene products being able to present antigens to T cells[13]. The extensive polymorphism at each locus thus has the potential to double the number of different MHC molecules[14] expressed in an individual and thereby increases the diversity already available through polygeny .

In addition to the highly polymorphic 'classical' MHC class I and class II genes, there are many genes encoding MHC class I-type molecules that show little polymorphism; most of these have yet to be assigned a function. They are linked to the class I region of the MHC and their exact number varies greatly between species and even between members of the same species. These genes have been termed MHC class IB[15] genes; like MHC class I genes, they encode β2-microglobulin-associated cell-surface molecules. Their expression on cells is variable, both in the amount expressed at the cell surface and in the tissue distribution "

In human, the main function of major histocompatibility complex (MHC) Class II molecules, is to present processed antigens which are derived primarily, from

---

[7] https://www.ncbi.nlm.nih.gov/books/n/imm/A2528/def-item/A2579/
[8] https://www.ncbi.nlm.nih.gov/books/n/imm/A2528/def-item/A3065/
[9] https://www.ncbi.nlm.nih.gov/books/n/imm/A2528/def-item/A2709/
[10] https://www.ncbi.nlm.nih.gov/books/n/imm/A2528/def-item/A2870/
[11] https://www.ncbi.nlm.nih.gov/books/n/imm/A2528/def-item/A3064/
[12] https://www.ncbi.nlm.nih.gov/books/n/imm/A2528/def-item/A2709/
[13] https://www.ncbi.nlm.nih.gov/books/n/imm/A2528/def-item/A3278/
[14] https://www.ncbi.nlm.nih.gov/books/n/imm/A2528/def-item/A3065/
[15] https://www.ncbi.nlm.nih.gov/books/n/imm/A2528/def-item/A3060/

exogeneous sources.

Constitutive expression of MHC Class II molecules, is also confined to professional antigen- presenting cells (APC) of the immune system (Ref.2)

Since we have discovered the IPA (Invertebrate Primitive Antibody)(Ref. 3,4,5,6), to acquire a better understanding of the invertebrate immune system , it seemed useful to look for MHC class I, class II genes in invertebrates with Ophiocomina nigra (Ophuirids), Antedon bifida (Crinoïds) as model of studies.

MATERIALS AND METHODS:

Animals: Ophiocomina nigra (Ophuirid) Antedon bifida(Crinoïd) were obtained at the station « Of Biologie Marine of Roscoff » France.

Obtention of ophuirid and crinoïd mRNA: Digestive coeca were excised from their bodies and

 mRNA were obtained from Uptizol (Interchim) then quality controls were operated. (Ref.7)

 Sequencing : Sequencing was made on Illumina Next Seq 500 with paired-end : 2. 75 bp

Transcriptome was assembled from RNA-Seq fastq files using Trinity v2.1.1 (Ref.8) with default parameters. A BLAST database was created with the assembled transcripts using makeblastdb application from ncbi-blast+ (v2.2.31+). The sequences of transcripts of interest were then blasted against this database using blastn application from ncbi-blast+ (Ref.9) with parameter word_size 7.

RESULTS:

First,it is shown a table in which are presented characteristics of HLA-E (MHC Class I)

HLA-DQB1 (MHC Class II) genes in Ophiocomina nigra (Ophuirids).Sequences are following

QueryID	Query Name	SubjectID	Identity (%)	Length	Mismatch	Gapopen	Query cover (%)	E-value	Bitscore
NM_005516.6	HLA-	TRINITY_DN6320_c0_g1_i1	78,63	117	22	2	4,00	2,00E-	75,00

	E									12	
NM_002123.4	HLA-DQB1	TRINITY_DN20883_c0_g1_i1	90,91	33	3		0		2,00	8,00E-04	45,40

>TRINITY_DN6320_c0_g1_i1 HLA-E
5'AGAGGACACGTCATTCTGAGCGTAAGGGCCGCAGCGAAAGGTGGCAGG
GCCCGCGCTTTT
AAAGGCTGAAATCCCGGCGGCTCAGGCCTGTCGTTTCCAGCACTTTGGGA
GGCCCAGGAA
GATGGATCGCTTGAGGCCAGGAGTTCGGGACTAGCCTGGCCAACATGGTG
AACACCCGTC
TCTACTAAAAATAGATCGGAAGAGCGTCGTGTT3'

>TRINITY_DN20883_c0_g1_i1 HLA-DQB1
5'GTAAAACAGCATTTCATCTGAAAAGAAATTCAATGTCCAAAGTTCAAAA
ACTCTGTGAAG
ACTTGAATGCAAAAAGTACTCAAGTCCATCACATATTTGGCATTTTTAGATA
TGATCTTC
CAAAGATTTTAAAATAAAACAAAAGAAAAACCAAAAGAAGAAAAAAATT
TAACAAAAAAA
TAAAGGGCCAAAAAAAATTTTAAAAAAAAAAAAAACCCCCATTTTTTTTGG
GTCTAAAAAA
AAAAAAAAAAAAAAAAATCGC3'

Two genes:HLA-E, HLA-B (ClassI) appear in the following table in Antedon bifida:

QueryID	Query Name	SubjectID	Identity (%)	Length	Mismatch	Gapopen	Query cover (%)	E-value	Bitscore
NM_005516.6	HLA-E	TRINITY_DN19334_c8_g2_i1	88,15	287	28	4	11,00	2,00E-91	337,00
NM_005514.8	HLA-B	TRINITY_DN15013_c0_g1_i1	100,00	21	0	0	1,00	3,70E-02	39,90

The sequences in 5'-3' follow:

>TRINITY_DN19334_c8_g2_i1 HLA-E
5'TGTAATCCCAGCACTTTGGGAGGCCGAGGCGGGCGGATCACGAGGTCAG
GAGATCGAGAC
CATCCTGGCTAACACAGTGAAACCCCGTCTCTACTAAAAATACAAAAAATT
AGCCGGGCG

TGGTGGCGGGCGCCTGTAGTCCCAGCTACTCGGGAGGCTGAGGCAGGAG
AATGGCGTGAA
CCCGGGAGGCGGAGCTTGCAGTGAGCCGAGATCGCGCCACTGCACTCCAG
CCTGGGCGAC
AGAGCGAGACTCTGTCTCAAAAAAAAAAAAAAAAAAAAAAAAAA3'

>TRINITY_DN15013_c0_g1_i1 HLA-B
5'GCCGAATATGATGCAGAGGTATCAGGGGGTGAAGCATCTGGAGGTGAGG
TATCGGCAGGA
GAGGCATCTGGGGGAGAAGCTGAACAATCTGACAATGAAAGCGATTAGAT
AACATTTTTT
TAATTCTAGTTGCAGCCTAAATATTTCGATATTACTTTTTTTTACTAGTTGAA
TGATTAA
CAAAAGAAAGCAACAACTGTGGTAATATTGCTAATTATGAAATGAAAAATG
TTTAATGTG
GCCCTGACACTAAATTGTAAACTGTTTTTTAGTAATAAGAATTTCAATAGCT
TCTCTGAA
AGAAGATGTCTCTGAGAGAGTAATATTTGACAGGTTCAGTGTATTTAAAGA
CTTATAATG
TAAAGCAGAGATGTAACTAGAGAAACCTAGATATTGATGTCAACAAACTAA
GGGTGCATG
GAAAATGTGAAAGACTTTAAGAGTGGGTGACCCTGCCTACCAACACAATT
CAATCCATGT
TTGAGGCTTTTTTTCATTAGCCTAATAGTGAAGTCAGTGGCGTAAGGCCCC
CTTGTTTAG
CACTCCTAAGGGTCCCTAATGATGGATAATTGTATTGGGCTCTTCATGCTCT
GGGGCCCT
GGGTTTAGCTAGTGAGTGCTCATAGCAGTTGGCTGGGCAAGGTTAGAAAG
CAATGGTTCT
GTGCAGACATTTGCATTTAATTGACCAATATTTCAAATCGTGTGTTACACAG
GAATCATA
ACCTAATCAGCAGTTGTTTTTAATAAACATTGCATCTTGGTCGACGTAATAT
TGTTATGG
ACTGTCTGTGAAACCATGTGAATCTAAACTCTTAAAAATGCCTGCCTCTCC
TGTCCTTGC
TAAATATAAATTTGTTTTCTCAATTAGGCG

GCCCTGACACTAAATTGTAAACTGTTTTTTAGTAATAAGAATTTCAATAGCT
TCTCTGAA
AGAAGATGTCTCTGAGAGAGTAATATTTGACAGGTTCAGTGTATTTAAAGA
CTTATAATG
TAAAGCAGAGATGTAACTAGAGAAACCTAGATATTGATGTCAACAAACTAA
GGGTGCATG
GAAAATGTGAAAGACTTTAAGAGTGGGTGACCCTGCCTACCAACACAATT
CAATCCATGT
TTGAGGCTTTTTTTCATTAGCCTAATAGTGAAGTCAGTGGCGTAAGGCCCC
CTTGTTTAG
CACTCCTAAGGGTCCCTAATGATGGATAATTGTATTGGGCTCTTCATGCTCT
GGGGCCCT
GGGTTTAGCTAGTGAGTGCTCATAGCAGTTGGCTGGGCAAGGTTAGAAAG
CAATGGTTCT
GTGCAGACATTTGCATTTAATTGACCAATATTTCAAATCGTGTGTTACACAG
GAATCATA
ACCTAATCAGCAGTTGTTTTTAATAAACATTGCATCTTGGTCGACGTAATAT
TGTTATGG
ACTGTCTGTGAAACCATGTGAATCTAAACTCTTAAAAATGCCTGCCTCTCC
TGTCCTTGC
TAAATATAAATTTGTTTTCTCAATTAGGCG

CONCLUSION:

MHC class I and classII genes exist in Echinodermata, at least in Echinodermata which possess a sophisticated immune system as Asterids, Ophuirids and Crinoïds. It would be interesting also to study MHC system in Echinodermata which present only innate immune response as Echinids, Holothurids (Ref.10)

The HLA-DQB1 gene is a part of a family of genes called the human leukocyte antigen (HLA) complex.

The found HLA-B gene and HLA-E gene belong also to the HLA complex (MHC Class I): it helps the immune system to distinguish the body own proteins from proteins made by foreign invaders such as viruses and bacteria (Ref. 11, 12, 13)

Although all efforts to find in Invertebrates a Major Histocompatibility Complex System have been unsuccessful, we find to day, for the first time, a MHC class II gene (HLA-DQB1 gene) a MHC class I (HLA-B HLA-E genes)in Echinodermata: It's of great novelty.It's a fundamental discovery in the domain of Comparative and Adaptative Immunology.

REFERENCES:

1)Janeway, C.A et al (2001) Immunobiology, New York Garland Science ed.

2) Holling , T.M et al (2004) Hum.Immunol 65(4) 282-90

3)Leclerc, M. (2018) Archives of Immunology and Allergy 1(2) 1-2

4) Leclerc, M. et al(2016) E.C Microbiology 3(5) 539-41

5) Leclerc, M et al (2016) E.C Microbiology 4(5) 759-60

6)Leclerc, M. et al (2018) Int. J.Vaccine Res 3(1) 1-2

7)Vincent, N. et al (2014) Meta Gene 2 320-22

8) Grabher, M.G et al (2011) Nature Biotechnology 29 644-52

9) Altschul, S.F et al (1990) J.Mol.Biol 215(3) 403-10

10)Leclerc,M. (2018) Int. J. Biotech. And Bioeng 5(1) 17-18

11)Hiby, S.E et al (2004) J. Exp. Med 200(8) 957-65

12)Khakoo, S.I (2004) Science 305 872-74

13) Nair, R.P et al (2006) AJHG 78(5) 827-51

NEW CYTOKINE GENES IN AN INVERTEBRATE: THROMBOXANE ONES IN ECHINODERMATA.EVIDENCE OF PLATELETS

By Michel Leclerc

Abstract: Two main points assert the existence of « platelets » in Echinodermata (Invertebtates): a)the evidence of thromboxane genes in an ophuirid, Ophiocomina nigra b)the appearance of T.E.M platelets, in the asterid, Asterias rubens. Opuirids and asterids(Echinodermata) possess each an IGKAPPA gene.

INTRODUCTION

The appearance of platelets, in Asterias rubens was just described (Ref.1 Fig 1) : They resemble blood platelets of vertebrates.

The aim of this work is to look for genes implicated in the initiation and synthesis of thromboxane which plays a rôle in platelet biochemistry (in vertebrates).

Thromboxane A synthetase gene, Thromboxane A2 receptor gene are the main genes which represent thromboxane activity in vertebrates. Thromboxane is also a cytokine, regulated by immune system and immune genes we research in the Ophiocomina nigra genome.

MATERIALS AND METHODS:

1) Ophiocomina nigra was purchased by the Laboratory of Roscoff (France). Digestive coeca were excised.RNA was extracted.

2a) Ophiocomina nigra and its preparation to obtain mRNA have already been described (Ref.2) .Furthermore quality controls were made.

2b) sequencing:

Transcriptome was assembled from RNA-Seq fastq files using Trinity v2.1.1 (Ref.3) with default parameters. A BLAST database was created with the assembled transcripts using makeblastdb application from ncbi-blast+ (v2.2.31+). The sequences of transcripts of interest were then blasted against this database using blastn application from ncbi-blast+ (Ref .4) with parameter word_size 7.

RESULTS

We observe a sea star Asterias rubens platelet in T.E.M (Ref.1, Fig.1)

25 Evidence of Platelets in Echinodermata

On the other hand, a table summarizes the genomic results. TBXA2R represents the human thromboxane A2 receptor gene, TBXAS1 the human synthetase on

Query ID	Query Name	Subject ID	Identity (%)	Length	Mismatch	Gapopen	Query cover	E-value	Bitscore
NM_001060.5	TBXA2R	TRINITY_DN38594_c0_g1_i1	77,93	222,00	34,00	9,00	13,00	2,00E-27	124,00
NM_001061.5	TBXAS1	TRINITY_DN22549_c0_g1_i1	84,21	38,00	6,00	0,00	2,00	1,60E-01	38,10

The sequences of the transcrriptomes are following: first TBXA2R one

>TRINITY_DN38594_c0_g1_i1

5'ATATATCATATATGATATAGTACCTTTGTTATATATCATAATACATATAAATGT
GTATTA
TGTTATCTATAATTATATAATTTCATATATAAGATGTATAATATGTATCATATATT
ATAT
ATGTTATGTAATATATATAGTATATATAAGATGACACAGGATAAATATTATATA
CTATGA
CATATAAAATATATGAGGTTATATGTTACATATAAGGCATAGCACATAACATG
TAATATA
TATCATATATAATTTTTTTTTTAGACAGAATCTTGTCCTGTTGCACAGGGTGGG
GTACAAT
GGCGCCATCTTTGCTCACTGCAACTTCTGCCTCACGGGTCCAAGCGATTGT
CCTCCCTCA
GCCTCCCAGGTAGCTGGGACTACACCACACTGGGACTACACCAGCTGCCA
CCATGCCTAG
CTAATTTTTGTATTTTTGGTAGAGACAGGGTTTTGCCGTGTTGCCCAGGCTG
GTAGATCG3'

Second TBAXS1 transcriptome :

>TRINITY_DN22549_c0_g1_i1

5'AAATAAGCATACGCATGGAAGAATCACTCAGATTTTTATGTTAAATAGGA
GGAACTTAGA
AAACACCAAGTGTGGATTTGGAGAATTTTGTAAAACTTAACCAAAGACAA

TGCCTAATCA
CATTGAGGGCAACATAAGTGGCACTATGTGTGTCATCGGCTCAACAGTTCA
TTCATCATC
ATCGGGATCTAACAAAATGACACATTGTAGGCATAATCATAACAGGACTCG
GCGTAGGTT
ATCAGCAACAGCTATGATTGGAGTACTCGGAGGA3'

DISCUSSION AND CONCLUSION:

Thromboxane A2 gene, we found in ophuirids(Echinodermata) induces a cytokine in human (Ref 5). Thromboxane A2 produced by activated platelets, has prothrombotic properties. It stimulates activation of new platelets as well as increases platelet aggregation (Ref.5)

Genomic results assert the evidence of a new cytokine in invertebrate: the thromboxane. Furthermore, TEM results (Ref.1 Fig.1) show structures which resemble blood platelets. In conclusion, it was clearly shown that platelets and thromboxane cytokine exist in Echinodermata: It's a great novelty in invertebrates !

26Evidence of Platelets in Echinodermata

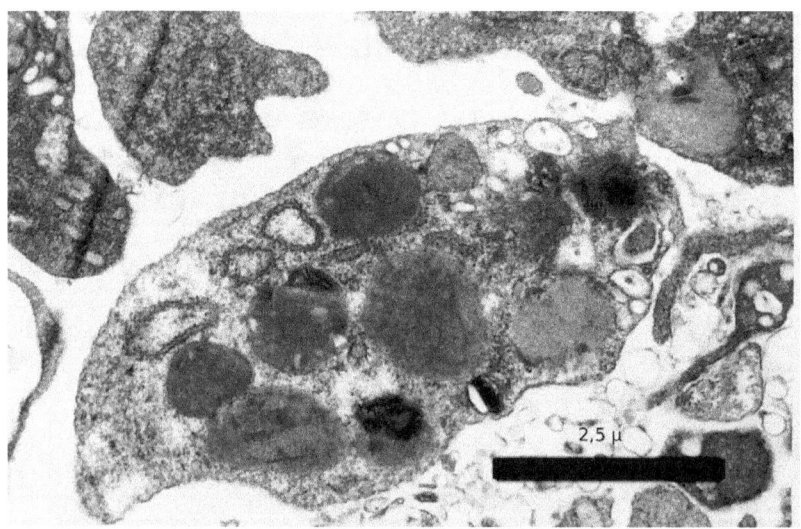

Figure 1

REFERENCES:

1)Leclerc M.(2019) « Platelet's problem in Echinodermata » IBBJ (2019) submitted

2) Leclerc M.   (2018) « A new gene in Ophiocomina nigra : An ophuirid Igkappa gene » J.Appl.Biotechnol. Bioeng. 5(5) : 303-304

3)Grabherr M.G,B.J Haas, M.Yassour, J.Z Levin, D.A Thompson, Ido Amit et al.l (2011) « Full-length transcriptome assembly from RNA-Seq data without a reference genome » Nature Biotechnology 29 : 644-652

4)Altschul S.F, W.Gish, W Miller, E.W Mijers and D.J Lipman (1990) « Basic local alignment search tool »   J. Mol.Biol 215 (3) : 403-410

5) Carter A.B, M.M Monick and G.W Hunninghake (1999)   « Both Erk and p38 kinases are necessary for cytokine gene transcription » Am.J.Respir.Cell. Mol. Biol. 20:751-758

BENCE-JONES PROTEIN, RAT IGG, H.R.P , ALKALINE PHOSPHATASE, BOVINE SERUM ALBUMINE(BSA) USED AS ANTIGENS IN THE IMMUNE RESPONSE OF THE SEA STAR.

by Michel Leclerc

556 rue Isabelle Romée, Sandillon (France)

Abstract: Immunocompetent cells were described in the sea star Asterina gibbosa: they recognize specifically various antigens. In the present work, Asterina gibbosa were immunized with Bence-Jones protein, others with BSA, other ones with Rat IGG, at last certain with H.RP (Horse-radish Peroxydase) and the last ones with Alkaline Phosphatase: a crossed immune reaction occurs between Rat IGG and B.J protein, but not between B.J and H.R.P not between Rat IGG and H.R.P , not between Alkaline Phosphatase and B.J, not between Alkaline Phosphatase and Rat IGG, and not between BSA and B.J or Alkaline Phosphatase used as antigens.

INTRODUCTION

Recently it was shown that immunized Asterina gibbosa (Asterids Echinodermata) to various proteins (Peroxydase; Alkalin phosphatase, Trypsin) shown specific immunocytochemical reactions in T.E.M (Ref ;1-2-3).

In the present study we attempt to estimate such reactions by the use of more sophisticated proteins: the Rat immunoglobulin IGG and Bence-Jones protein(Light chain of immunoglobulins produced by human myeloma) in comparison to H.R.P (Horse -radish Peroxydase).

MATERIALS AND METHODS

1)Sea stars: Asterina gibbosa were kept in aquarium , at 10° C, in running sea water.

2)Methods:

100 μg of HRP (Sigma Products) were injected in 5 Asterina gibbosa each: they were kept in a control aquarium. 7 days after the first injection, they were injected a second time with the same quantity of HRP, always in the coelomic cavity of each animal. They were placed in aquarium I .

A same experiment was done with Alkaline phosphatase (Sigma Products): 100 μg were injected in 5 Asterina gibbosa which were placed after in aquarium II.

A second injection was performed as precedently.

In the same time, 100 µl of a solution at 1mg/ml of Bence-Jones (BJ) protein were injected to 5 other Asterina gibbosa each, twice, like in the first experiment. They were placed in an aquarium III.

On the other hand, 100 µl of a Rat IGG solution at 1mg/ml were injected to 5 other Asterina gibbosa, placed in an other aquarium IV with running sea water as precedently.

At last 5 Asterina gibbosa were injected with 100µg each of Bovine Serum Albumine (Pentex) in aquarium V.

4 days after the last injection, all axial organs (AO) (Ref.3) were excised and fixed separately in glutaraldehyde (1,5% in cacodylate buffer) then rinsed in the same buffer.

Incubation in antigenic solution (Rat IGG coupled to peroxydase -Sigma Products) were performed, for each animal of Aquarium I, II, III, IV.V

A new fixation at glutaraldehyde of 10 minutes occur for all AO (1 % in cacodylate buffer).

AO were rinced in cacodylate buffer then treated with diaminobenzidine (Ref.3) at last dehydrated (Alcohol 70 to Alcohol 100°) and finally embedded in Epon.

Incubation in Rat IGG coupled to peroxydase was also performed for each animal of Aquarium I,II,III, IV,V.Following steps have been precedently described.

Incubation in HRP was done for also each animal of Aquarium I, II, III, IV,V.Following steps are now well-known (Ref.3)

At last incubation in antigenic solution of Alkaline Phosphatase was realized fo each animal of Aquarium I, II, III, IV, V. Following steps have already been described.(Ref.3)

Cuts were done with a LKB ultrotome. Observations in TEM were realized with a Hitachi Microscope.

RESULTS

Immuunolabelling was seen in treated animals either with Rat IGG, Bence-Jones protein , HRP, Alkaline phosphatase, BSA antigens.

These labelling are situated at the level of perinuclear space (EP) next to Nucleus (N) Reticulum endoplasmic (RE) Golgi apparatus (G) and Lysosomes (L) of the sea star plasmolymphocytes in TEM as previously described (Table.1): Labelling with HRP.

DISCUSSION CONCLUSION

1) Labelling occurs in treated animals to Rat IGG, Bence-Jones protein, HRP, Alkaline phosphatase Bovine Serum Albumine (BSA) antigens.

2) It is noticeable that sea star Immune system makes no differences between Rat

IGG and BJ protein antigens: there is a CROSSED reaction. BUT:

3)There is no crossed reactions, between HRP and BJ protein, between Alkaline phosphatase and BJ protein

4)There is no crossed reactions between Rat IGG and HRP, between Rat IGG and Alkaline phosphatase

5) The sea star recognizes specifically HRP from Phosphatase alkaline, from Bovine Serum Albumine (BSA) (Ref.3) and vice versa.

We retain that Asterina gibbosa is able to recognize many antigens but not all the antigens the man does: it must be claimed.

References

1) Leclerc, M (2020) ejbio 1.4.61
2) Leclerc, M (2020) J.viro.res.rep 1(1) 1-2
3) Leclerc, M (1973) Ann. Immunol Inst. Pasreur 124C: 363-74

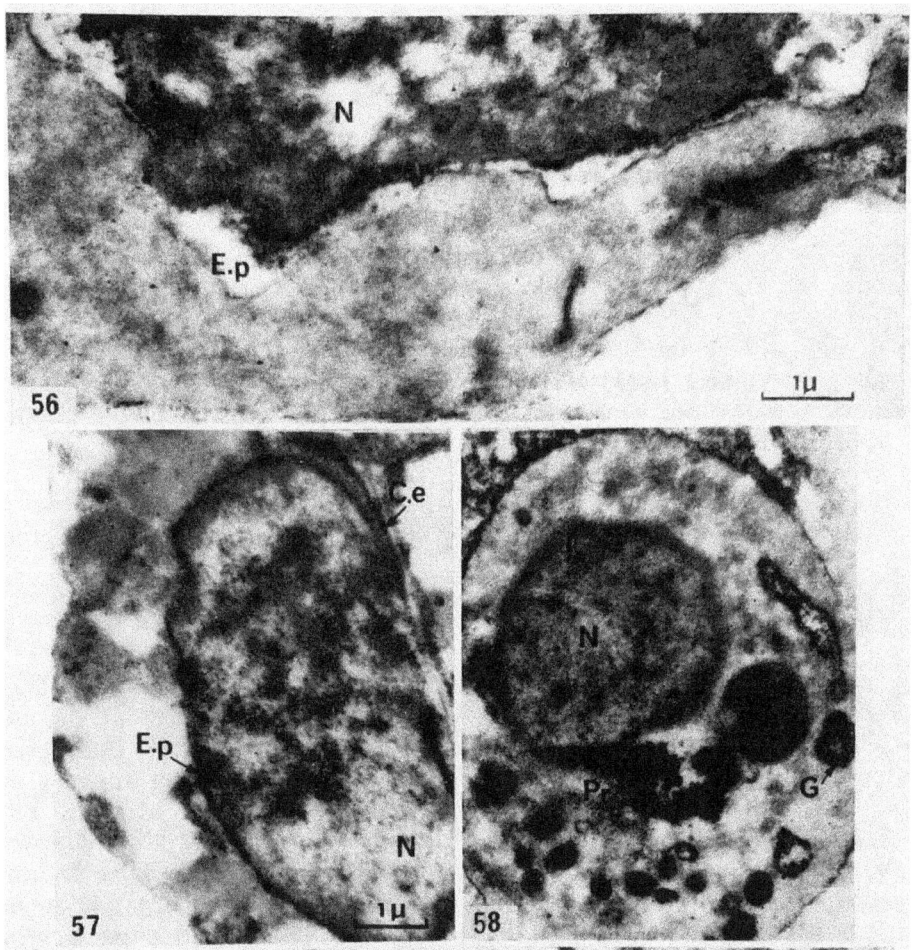

TABLE I: IMMUNOENZYMATIC REACTIONS IN ASTERINA GIBBOSA (REF 3) LABELLING WITH HRP AS ANTIGEN.

Publisher: Eliva Press SRL

Email: info@elivapress.com

Eliva Press is an independent publishing house established for the publication and dissemination of academic works all over the world. Company provides high quality and professional service for all of our authors.

Our Services:
Free of charge, open-minded, eco-friendly, innovational.

-Free standard publishing services (manuscript review, step-by-step book preparation, publication, distribution, and marketing).
-No financial risk. The author is not obliged to pay any hidden fees for publication.
-Editors. Dedicated editors will assist step by step through the projects.
-Money paid to the author for every book sold. Up to 50% royalties guaranteed.
-ISBN (International Standard Book Number). We assign a unique ISBN to every Eliva Press book.
-Digital archive storage. Books will be available online for a long time. We don't need to have a stock of our titles. No unsold copies. Eliva Press uses environment friendly print on demand technology that limits the needs of publishing business. We care about environment and share these principles with our customers.
-Cover design. Cover art is designed by a professional designer.
-Worldwide distribution. We continue expanding our distribution channels to make sure that all readers have access to our books.

www.elivapress.com